# From Fear to Faith

## *Conquering Anxiety with Spiritual Strength*

*by*

## Kristine Hawkins

# Table of Contents

# Introduction: The Journey from Darkness to Light

## Opening Reflection

Anxiety and fear have a way of creeping into our lives when we least expect it. They can paralyze us, keeping us from living fully and freely. Perhaps you know this all too well. Maybe you've felt the weight of fear pressing down on your chest, the unease of anxiety stealing your peace and robbing you of joy. I've been there too, and I know how overwhelming it can be. But I also know that there is hope—a way out of the darkness and into the light.

**Purpose of the Book**

This book is a guide for those who find themselves trapped in the shadows of fear and anxiety, longing for a way out but unsure where to turn. It's for the person who wants to move from a place of fear to a place of faith, where anxiety no longer holds power over them. Through spiritual insights, scripture, and practical techniques, this book will help you embark on a journey toward peace, guided by the light of faith.

You'll discover how to anchor yourself in spiritual strength, finding the courage to face your fears and the serenity to trust in something greater than yourself. Whether you're just beginning your journey or have been walking this path for some time, my hope is that this book will provide you with the tools and inspiration you need to overcome anxiety and embrace a life filled with faith and peace.

**The Analogy: From Darkness to Light**

In the pages that follow, we'll explore the journey from darkness to light—a journey from the oppressive weight of fear to the liberating embrace of faith. Imagine anxiety as a dark cloud that obscures your vision, making it difficult to see the path ahead. Now, imagine faith as a bright, guiding light that cuts through the darkness, illuminating your way and offering warmth, hope, and direction.

This analogy will serve as our compass throughout the book, reminding us that no matter how deep the darkness may seem, there is always light waiting to break through. With each chapter, you'll be guided closer to that light, learning how to harness spiritual strength to conquer your fears and find lasting peace.

In the next chapters, we'll dive deeper into understanding the nature of anxiety and fear, and how they can be overcome through faith. You'll learn practical techniques for navigating life's challenges with the confidence that comes from knowing you're guided by the light of God's love and wisdom.

**A Personal Invitation**

As you begin this journey, I invite you to open your heart to the possibility of transformation. Know that you are not alone—many have walked this path before you, and many are walking it now. Together, we will explore the power of faith to conquer fear and the ways in which spiritual strength can light your way to peace. Let this book be a companion on your journey, offering encouragement, insight, and

the reassurance that light will always overcome
darkness.

Let's begin this journey together, moving from fear
to faith, and from anxiety to peace. The light is
waiting to guide you.

## Chapter 1: The Darkness of Fear

**Understanding Anxiety**

Anxiety is a complex and often misunderstood
emotion. It's more than just feeling nervous before
a big event or worrying about an upcoming
challenge. For many, anxiety is a constant
companion, an unwelcome guest that lingers in the

background, whispering fears and doubts that disrupt daily life. Anxiety can manifest in various ways—physically, emotionally, and spiritually. It can cause your heart to race, your thoughts to spiral, and your spirit to feel heavy.

The roots of anxiety can be deep, often intertwined with past experiences, unhealed wounds, and fears of the unknown. Sometimes it's triggered by a specific event, but other times it seems to arise out of nowhere, leaving you feeling helpless and overwhelmed. In these moments, it's easy to feel trapped in the darkness, unsure of how to find your way out.

**The Grip of Fear**

Fear, like anxiety, can be paralyzing. It tells us that we're not safe, that we're not capable, that something terrible is just around the corner. Fear can keep us from stepping out in faith, from pursuing our dreams, from living the life we're meant to live. It whispers lies that we start to believe, lies that say we're not good enough, that we'll fail, that we'll be hurt.

The grip of fear can be strong, holding us back from the fullness of life that God intends for us. It can make the world seem like a dangerous place, where every step is fraught with peril. When fear takes hold, it's easy to withdraw, to shrink back, and to let anxiety rule our lives. But that's not the life we're called to live.

## Biblical Perspectives on Fear and Anxiety

The Bible speaks often about fear and anxiety, acknowledging these emotions as part of the human experience but also offering a path to overcome them. One of the most repeated commands in the Bible is "Do not be afraid." This is not a command to suppress or ignore fear but an invitation to trust in God, who is greater than our fears.

Consider these words from Isaiah 41:10: "So do not fear, for I am with you; do not be dismayed, for I am your God. I will strengthen you and help you; I will uphold you with my righteous right hand." Here, we see a powerful reminder that we are not alone in our fears. God promises to be with us, to strengthen and support us, even in the darkest times.

Philippians 4:6-7 offers further encouragement: "Do not be anxious about anything, but in every situation, by prayer and petition, with thanksgiving, present your requests to God. And the peace of God, which transcends all understanding, will guard your hearts and your minds in Christ Jesus." This passage invites us to bring our anxieties to God, trusting that His peace—a peace beyond human understanding—will guard us.

These scriptures, and many others, provide a foundation for overcoming fear and anxiety through faith. They remind us that while fear is real, it doesn't have to control us. With God's help, we can find the strength to move forward, to step out of the darkness and into the light.

**The Invitation to Overcome**

As we begin this journey, it's important to acknowledge where you are right now. Maybe you're feeling overwhelmed by anxiety, burdened by fears that you can't seem to shake. Perhaps you've tried to overcome these struggles on your own, only to find yourself back in the same place, feeling defeated. But there is hope.

This chapter is an invitation to explore the nature of your fears and anxieties, to understand where they come from and how they've been affecting your life. It's also an invitation to begin the process of overcoming them, not through your own strength, but by turning to the light of faith. You don't have to walk this path alone—God is with you, ready to guide you every step of the way.

As we move forward, we'll explore practical ways to confront fear and anxiety, using spiritual strength as our guide. We'll look at the tools and techniques that can help you break free from the darkness and embrace the light of faith. Remember, the journey from fear to faith is not an overnight transformation, but a gradual process of growth and healing. And it begins with understanding—understanding what fear and anxiety are, and understanding that with God's help, they can be overcome.

Let's take the first step together.

# Chapter 2: The Roots of Anxiety

**Identifying Triggers**

Anxiety often seems to come out of nowhere, striking when we least expect it. But if we look closer, we can often identify specific triggers— situations, thoughts, or memories that ignite the flame of anxiety within us. These triggers can be different for everyone; for some, it might be the fear of failure, while for others, it could be the anticipation of conflict or uncertainty about the future.

Identifying your triggers is a crucial step in overcoming anxiety. When you know what sets off your anxious thoughts, you can begin to prepare yourself spiritually and emotionally to face them. Journaling can be a powerful tool in this process. Take some time to reflect and write down situations or thoughts that seem to precede your anxiety. Notice any patterns that emerge, and consider how these triggers relate to deeper fears or unresolved issues.

By recognizing your triggers, you can start to address them directly, rather than being caught off guard. This awareness is the first step in diffusing their power over you.

**The Influence of the Past**

Our past experiences have a profound impact on how we view the world and respond to stressors.

Often, anxiety is rooted in unresolved pain, trauma, or negative experiences from the past. These memories can leave lasting imprints on our minds and hearts, influencing how we react to current situations.

Consider whether your anxiety might be tied to past experiences. Perhaps a painful relationship, a traumatic event, or even a pattern of negative thinking established in childhood has contributed to the way you experience anxiety today. Understanding the influence of the past can bring clarity and help you see that your anxiety is not just about the present—it's often about how the present interacts with unresolved issues from the past.

In this chapter, it's important to acknowledge that healing from past wounds is a process. It may require time, patience, and sometimes professional support. But as you bring these issues into the light of faith, you'll find that God's love and healing can begin to transform even the deepest wounds.

**Generational Patterns**

Anxiety can also be influenced by generational patterns—behaviors, beliefs, and fears passed down from one generation to the next. These patterns can be subtle, embedded in the way we were raised or the environments we grew up in. Perhaps you've noticed that anxiety runs in your family, or that certain fears seem to be shared across generations.

Recognizing generational patterns can be both challenging and liberating. It's challenging because it requires us to confront the possibility that we've inherited not just physical traits but emotional and spiritual ones as well. But it's liberating because it gives us the opportunity to break the cycle, to choose a different path for ourselves and for future generations.

As you reflect on your own experiences, consider whether there are any generational patterns at play. Are there fears or anxieties that seem to have been passed down to you? How have these influenced your life, and what can you do to break free from them?

**Breaking the Cycle with Faith**

Once you've identified your triggers, understood the influence of the past, and recognized any generational patterns, the next step is to break the cycle. This is where faith plays a crucial role. The Bible offers many examples of individuals who, with God's help, broke free from the chains of fear, doubt, and anxiety.

In 2 Timothy 1:7, we are reminded: "For God has not given us a spirit of fear, but of power and of love and of a sound mind." This verse serves as a powerful declaration that fear and anxiety do not come from God; instead, He gives us the strength to overcome them.

To break the cycle of anxiety, it's essential to lean into your faith, trusting that God will provide the strength, wisdom, and peace you need. This might involve daily practices of prayer, meditation on scripture, and surrounding yourself with a supportive community of believers who can encourage you on your journey.

Breaking the cycle also requires a commitment to renewal—a renewal of your mind, heart, and spirit. Romans 12:2 encourages us to be "transformed by the renewing of your mind." This renewal process involves replacing anxious thoughts with the truth of God's Word, choosing faith over fear, and allowing God's light to shine into the darkest corners of your life.

**Reflection and Preparation**

As we conclude this chapter, take some time to reflect on the roots of your anxiety. Consider the triggers, past experiences, and generational patterns that may be contributing to your current struggles. Write down your thoughts, and bring them before God in prayer, asking for His guidance and healing.

Remember, this is not a journey you have to take alone. God is with you, ready to lead you out of the darkness and into the light. The process of breaking free from anxiety may be gradual, but with each step you take in faith, you're moving closer to the peace that surpasses all understanding.

In the next chapter, we'll explore how to find the light that begins to shine through the darkness, offering hope and a way forward.

## Chapter 3: The Light Begins to Shine

**Awakening to Faith**

As you start to understand the roots of your anxiety, you may begin to feel a stirring of hope—a sense that there is a way out of the darkness. This hope is the first glimmer of light, an awakening to the possibility of living a life guided by faith rather than ruled by fear.

Faith is not just a vague belief in something greater; it's a living, active trust in God's love, wisdom, and power. It's the assurance that even in the midst of your deepest fears, you are not alone. God is with you, ready to lead you out of anxiety's grip and into a place of peace.

This chapter is about cultivating that faith—nurturing the light that has begun to shine in your heart. It's about learning to trust in God's presence and promises, even when fear tries to cloud your vision.

## The Role of Prayer

Prayer is one of the most powerful tools we have in the fight against anxiety. It's not just a ritual or a last resort; it's a direct line of communication with the Creator of the universe, who cares deeply about every detail of your life. Through prayer, you can bring your fears, worries, and anxieties to God, trusting that He hears you and will respond with love and compassion.

In Philippians 4:6-7, we're encouraged: "Do not be anxious about anything, but in every situation, by prayer and petition, with thanksgiving, present your requests to God. And the peace of God, which transcends all understanding, will guard your hearts and your minds in Christ Jesus."

This scripture reminds us that prayer is not just about asking for help; it's also about giving thanks. When you focus on gratitude, you shift your perspective away from fear and toward the goodness of God. This shift can be incredibly powerful in calming your mind and heart.

Consider setting aside time each day for prayer, making it a regular part of your routine. Use this time to pour out your heart to God, sharing your fears and anxieties, and asking for His guidance and peace. You might also find it helpful to keep a prayer journal, where you can write down your prayers and reflect on how God answers them over time.

**Scripture as a Beacon**

Just as a lighthouse guides ships safely to shore, scripture can guide you through the storms of life. The Bible is filled with promises, encouragement, and wisdom that can help you navigate the challenges of anxiety. By meditating on scripture, you can replace the lies of fear with the truth of God's Word.

One powerful verse to meditate on is Isaiah 26:3: "You will keep in perfect peace those whose minds are steadfast, because they trust in you." This verse reminds us that peace is possible when we keep our minds focused on God and trust in His plans.

Another key verse is Psalm 34:4: "I sought the Lord, and he answered me; he delivered me from all my fears." This scripture offers hope that when we seek God, He will respond and deliver us from our fears.

Make a habit of reading and meditating on scripture daily. Choose verses that resonate with you, and memorize them so that you can call on them in moments of anxiety. Let these verses be a beacon of light, guiding you back to faith when fear threatens to overwhelm you.

**Personal Reflection**

As you begin to awaken to faith and embrace the light of God's presence, take some time for personal reflection. Consider how your relationship with God has influenced your experience of anxiety. Have there been moments when faith helped you overcome fear? Are there areas of your life where you struggle to trust God fully?

Reflecting on these questions can help you identify areas where you need to grow in faith and trust. It can also help you recognize the progress you've already made, giving you encouragement to continue on the journey.

You might find it helpful to write down your reflections in a journal, noting any insights or revelations that come to you. This process of self-examination can be a valuable tool in deepening your faith and strengthening your resolve to overcome anxiety.

**A New Path Forward**

As the light of faith begins to shine in your life, you'll start to see a new path forward—one that leads away from the darkness of anxiety and toward the peace of God. This path may not always be easy, and there will likely be challenges along the way. But as you continue to cultivate your faith, you'll find that the light grows brighter, guiding you with increasing clarity.

In the next chapter, we'll explore how to stay on this path, using spiritual practices and community support to strengthen your faith and maintain your focus on the light. Remember, this journey is a process, and every step you take in faith brings you closer to the peace that God promises.

**Chapter 4: Guided by the Light**

## Walking with God

As you continue your journey from fear to faith, it's essential to recognize that this journey is not one you undertake alone. God walks with you every step of the way, offering guidance, comfort, and strength. Walking with God means inviting Him into every aspect of your life, allowing His presence to influence your thoughts, decisions, and actions.

Walking with God requires a conscious choice to trust Him, even when the path ahead is unclear. Proverbs 3:5-6 encourages us: "Trust in the Lord with all your heart and lean not on your own understanding; in all your ways submit to him, and he will make your paths straight." This passage reminds us that God's wisdom far exceeds our own, and when we lean on Him, He will guide us along the right path.

This daily walk with God involves both big decisions and small moments. It's about turning to Him when anxiety starts to creep in, asking for His peace and guidance. It's about seeking His will in your decisions, trusting that He knows what's best for you. And it's about remembering that you are never alone—He is always with you, lighting your way.

**Spiritual Practices for Daily Life**

To walk closely with God and remain guided by His light, it's helpful to cultivate spiritual practices that keep you grounded in faith. These practices serve as daily reminders of God's presence and power, helping you to stay focused on Him rather than on your fears.

1. **Daily Prayer**: Set aside time each day to connect with God in prayer. Use this time to share your concerns, seek His guidance, and express your gratitude. Prayer helps you to center your thoughts on God and invites His peace into your heart.

2. **Scripture Reading and Meditation**: Regularly read and meditate on God's Word. Let scripture fill your mind and heart, offering encouragement and wisdom. Choose passages that speak to your current

struggles, and reflect on how they apply to your life.

3.  **Worship**: Engaging in worship—whether through music, singing, or simply praising God in your thoughts—helps to lift your spirit and refocus your mind on His goodness. Worship reminds you of God's greatness and helps to diminish the power of fear.

4.  **Gratitude Journaling**: Keeping a gratitude journal is a powerful way to shift your focus from anxiety to thankfulness. Each day, write down a few things you are grateful for, no matter how small. This practice can help you to see the positive in your life and recognize God's blessings.

5.  **Mindful Presence**: Practice being fully present in the moment, mindful of God's presence with you. When anxiety arises, take a moment to breathe deeply, acknowledge God's nearness, and let go of the worries that threaten to overwhelm you.

## The Power of Community

While your personal relationship with God is central to overcoming anxiety, the support of a faith-filled community can also be incredibly valuable. Being part of a community of believers offers encouragement, accountability, and shared wisdom. When you surround yourself with others who are also walking in faith, you gain strength from their experiences and insights.

1.  **Joining a Faith Community**: Whether it's a
    church, a small group, or a Bible study,
    being part of a faith community provides
    you with a network of support. These
    connections allow you to share your
    journey, receive prayer, and grow in your
    faith alongside others.

2.  **Sharing Your Story**: Don't be afraid to
    share your struggles with trusted members
    of your community. Opening up about your
    anxieties can be freeing, and it allows others
    to come alongside you in prayer and
    support. Your story might also encourage
    someone else who is facing similar
    challenges.

3. **Seeking Counsel**: Sometimes, anxiety can feel overwhelming, and professional or pastoral counseling may be beneficial. A counselor or pastor can provide you with additional tools and perspectives to help you navigate your journey from fear to faith.

4. **Serving Others**: Engaging in acts of service can be a powerful antidote to anxiety. When you focus on helping others, you shift your attention away from your fears and toward making a positive impact. Serving also allows you to experience the joy and fulfillment that comes from living out your faith.

**Real-Life Testimonies**

Hearing the testimonies of others who have overcome anxiety through faith can be incredibly inspiring and reassuring. Their stories serve as reminders that God is faithful and that He can bring you through even the darkest times.

Consider reading or listening to testimonies of those who have experienced God's light in the midst of their struggles. You might find these stories in books, podcasts, or through conversations with people in your community. As you hear how others have moved from fear to faith, let their experiences strengthen your resolve to continue your journey.

**Reflection and Commitment**

At this point in your journey, take some time to reflect on how you've been guided by God's light so far. What spiritual practices have been most helpful to you? How has being part of a faith community supported you? Are there areas where you still struggle to trust God fully?

Commit to deepening your walk with God, using the practices and support systems that resonate most with you. Remember that this journey is ongoing, and each day offers new opportunities to grow in faith and trust.

In the next chapter, we'll explore the obstacles that can arise on this path and how to overcome them with God's help. As you continue to walk in His light, know that He is leading you toward a life of peace, free from the grip of anxiety.

## Chapter 5: Trusting in God's Timing

### The Patience of Faith

One of the most challenging aspects of overcoming anxiety is learning to trust in God's timing. We live in a world that values quick fixes and immediate results, but God often works on a different timeline. When we're in the midst of anxiety, it's natural to want relief as soon as possible. We pray, we seek, and we hope for an immediate change. But sometimes, God's answer requires us to wait, to be patient, and to trust that His timing is perfect.

Patience is a virtue that is closely tied to faith. It's about believing that God's plans are good, even when they don't align with our own desires or schedules. Psalm 27:14 encourages us: "Wait for the Lord; be strong and take heart and wait for the Lord." This waiting is not passive; it's an active, faith-filled waiting that involves trusting that God is working, even when we can't see it.

When anxiety pushes you to seek quick solutions, remind yourself that God's timing is always for your ultimate good. He sees the bigger picture and knows what you need, when you need it. Trusting in His timing means surrendering your own agenda and allowing Him to work in His way and in His time.

**Surrendering Control**

Anxiety often stems from a desire to control the uncontrollable. We want to manage outcomes, avoid uncertainties, and ensure that everything goes according to plan. But life doesn't work that way, and neither does faith. At its core, faith involves surrendering control to God, trusting that He is in charge and that His plans are better than anything we could orchestrate.

Proverbs 16:9 reminds us: "In their hearts humans plan their course, but the Lord establishes their steps." This verse encourages us to make plans, but ultimately to trust that God will guide our steps. Surrendering control doesn't mean giving up; it means handing over the reins to the One who knows the path ahead better than we do.

When you find yourself overwhelmed by anxiety, take a moment to acknowledge your desire for control. Then, consciously release that control to God. Pray for the strength to trust Him, even when the future feels uncertain. Remember that God is sovereign, and He is fully capable of handling whatever you're facing.

**Waiting with Hope**

Waiting on God's timing can be difficult, especially when you're anxious for change. But waiting doesn't have to be a time of despair. Instead, it can be a time of hope and expectation. When you wait with hope, you're actively trusting that God is working behind the scenes, preparing you for what's to come.

Isaiah 40:31 offers a powerful promise: "But those who hope in the Lord will renew their strength. They will soar on wings like eagles; they will run and not grow weary, they will walk and not be faint." This verse reminds us that hope is not passive; it is an active trust in God that brings renewal and strength. When we place our hope in the Lord, we are empowered to endure the waiting period with grace and patience.

During this time, consider what God might be teaching you. Perhaps He is building your character, deepening your faith, or preparing you for something greater than you can imagine. Waiting with hope involves a shift in perspective—from focusing on what we lack to trusting in what God is doing. It's about believing that God's timing is perfect and that His plans for you are good.

**Scriptures to Strengthen Your Trust**

As you navigate the challenges of waiting on God's timing, turning to scripture can provide comfort and encouragement. Here are some key verses to meditate on:

1. **Psalm 37:7**: "Be still before the Lord and wait patiently for him; do not fret when people succeed in their ways, when they carry out their wicked schemes." This verse encourages us to remain calm and patient, trusting that God's justice and timing will prevail.

2. **Lamentations 3:25-26**: "The Lord is good to those whose hope is in him, to the one who seeks him; it is good to wait quietly for the salvation of the Lord." These verses remind us that waiting on the Lord is good, and it is a practice that draws us closer to His goodness.

3. **Romans 8:25**: "But if we hope for what we do not yet have, we wait for it patiently."

This verse emphasizes the importance of patience in the process of hope, reinforcing the idea that faith involves trusting in what is not yet seen.

**Reflection and Application**

As you reflect on this chapter, consider the areas of your life where you are struggling with anxiety related to timing. Are there situations where you feel impatient, where you want God to act more quickly? Take time to write down these areas and bring them before God in prayer.

Ask God to help you trust in His timing, to surrender control, and to wait with hope. Reflect on the scriptures provided, and allow them to speak to your heart. Remember that God's timing is not just about delaying; it's about perfecting—perfecting your character, your faith, and His plan for your life.

In the next chapter, we'll explore the obstacles that can arise on this path and how to overcome them with God's help. As you continue to trust in His timing, know that He is leading you toward a future filled with His peace and purpose.

**Chapter 6: Overcoming Obstacles on the Path**

## Dealing with Doubt

As you journey from fear to faith, doubt is an obstacle that will inevitably arise. Doubt can manifest as questions about God's presence, uncertainty about His promises, or feelings of inadequacy in your own faith. It's important to understand that doubt is a natural part of the faith journey—it doesn't mean that your faith is weak or that you're failing.

Even some of the most faithful figures in the Bible experienced doubt. Consider Thomas, one of Jesus' disciples, who struggled to believe in the resurrection until he saw Jesus for himself (John 20:24-29). Jesus didn't condemn Thomas for his doubt; instead, He gently invited him to believe.

This shows us that God is not afraid of our doubts. He invites us to bring them to Him, to seek answers, and to trust in His faithfulness even when we can't see the full picture.

When you encounter doubt, approach it with honesty and bring it before God in prayer. Ask for His help in overcoming your doubts, and seek wisdom in scripture and through conversations with trusted spiritual mentors. Remember that doubt can be an opportunity for growth—it pushes you to seek deeper understanding and stronger faith.

**Resisting the Darkness**

Anxiety can often feel like a dark cloud that hovers over your life, making it difficult to see the light of faith. Even after making progress on your journey, there may be times when this darkness tries to return, threatening to pull you back into fear and despair.

Resisting this darkness requires vigilance and a firm commitment to your spiritual practices. Ephesians 6:11 reminds us to "put on the full armor of God, so that you can take your stand against the devil's schemes." This armor includes truth, righteousness, the gospel of peace, faith, salvation, the Word of God, and prayer. Each of these elements is crucial in defending against the attacks of anxiety and fear.

When you feel the darkness creeping in, turn immediately to prayer. Speak scriptures aloud, declaring God's promises over your life. Surround yourself with the support of your faith community, and don't hesitate to reach out for help. The darkness may be persistent, but the light of God is always stronger. By staying rooted in faith, you can resist the pull of anxiety and continue moving forward in peace.

**Scripture for Strength**

God's Word is a powerful tool in overcoming obstacles on your journey from fear to faith. When you feel weak, uncertain, or overwhelmed, turn to these scriptures for strength and encouragement:

1. **Isaiah 41:10**: "So do not fear, for I am with you; do not be dismayed, for I am your God. I will strengthen you and help you; I will

uphold you with my righteous right hand."
This verse is a reminder that God is always
with you, ready to give you the strength you
need to face any challenge.

2. **Psalm 46:1**: "God is our refuge and
strength, an ever-present help in trouble." In
times of trouble, you can find refuge and
strength in God, knowing that He is always
there to support you.

3. **Joshua 1:9**: "Have I not commanded you?
Be strong and courageous. Do not be afraid;
do not be discouraged, for the Lord your
God will be with you wherever you go."
This verse encourages you to be strong and
courageous, knowing that God's presence
goes with you in every situation.

**Reflection Questions**

As you reflect on this chapter, consider the following questions to help you identify and overcome the obstacles on your path:

1. **What doubts have you encountered on your journey from fear to faith? How have you addressed these doubts?**

2. **When has the darkness of anxiety tried to return, and how have you resisted it?**

3. **Which scriptures have brought you strength in times of weakness? How can you incorporate them more regularly into your spiritual practice?**

Take time to write down your reflections and bring them before God in prayer. Acknowledge the obstacles you've faced and ask for His continued guidance and strength as you move forward.

In the next chapter, we'll explore the power of forgiveness—both for others and for yourself—and how it plays a crucial role in freeing you from anxiety and leading you into deeper faith. As you continue to overcome the obstacles in your path, know that each step brings you closer to the peace and freedom that God desires for you.

## Chapter 7: The Power of Forgiveness

**Forgiving Others**

Forgiveness is a fundamental aspect of the Christian faith, and it plays a crucial role in overcoming anxiety. Holding onto resentment, anger, or bitterness can create a heavy burden on your heart, often fueling anxiety and preventing you from experiencing the peace that God desires for you. Forgiveness, however, is not just about releasing others from their wrongs; it's also about freeing yourself from the chains that bind you to the past.

In Matthew 6:14-15, Jesus teaches us, "For if you forgive other people when they sin against you, your heavenly Father will also forgive you. But if you do not forgive others their sins, your Father will not forgive your sins." This scripture underscores

the importance of forgiveness in our spiritual lives.
Forgiving others is not optional; it is essential for
our own spiritual well-being and our relationship
with God.

Forgiveness can be difficult, especially when the
hurt is deep. It doesn't mean that you condone the
wrong or that you forget the pain; rather, it means
that you choose to let go of the bitterness and anger,
leaving the judgment to God. It's a conscious
decision to release the hold that the offense has over
you, trusting that God will heal your wounds and
bring justice in His own time.

As you reflect on your journey, consider if there are
any people you need to forgive. Ask God to help
you in this process, to soften your heart, and to give

you the strength to let go of any lingering resentment. Remember that forgiveness is a process, and it may take time, but each step you take brings you closer to freedom and peace.

**Forgiving Yourself**

Just as it is important to forgive others, it is equally crucial to forgive yourself. Many people struggle with self-forgiveness, holding onto guilt, shame, or regret over past mistakes. These feelings can be a significant source of anxiety, weighing you down and preventing you from moving forward in faith.

The Bible assures us that God's forgiveness is complete. In 1 John 1:9, we read, "If we confess our sins, he is faithful and just and will forgive us our sins and purify us from all unrighteousness." When you bring your sins and mistakes before God, He is faithful to forgive you and cleanse you from all unrighteousness. If God, in His infinite love and mercy, has forgiven you, then you must also learn to forgive yourself.

Self-forgiveness requires grace—grace that comes from understanding that you are human, that you make mistakes, and that those mistakes do not define you. It's about accepting God's forgiveness and allowing His love to heal your heart. When you forgive yourself, you release the hold that guilt and shame have over your life, opening the door to peace and spiritual growth.

Take some time to reflect on any areas where you may be holding onto self-condemnation. Ask God to help you see yourself through His eyes—loved, forgiven, and redeemed. Let go of the past and embrace the new life that God offers you, free from the burden of guilt.

**The Biblical Call to Forgive**

The call to forgive is woven throughout the Bible, not just as a command but as an invitation to live a life of freedom and peace. In Colossians 3:13, we are reminded, "Bear with each other and forgive one another if any of you has a grievance against someone. Forgive as the Lord forgave you." This verse highlights that forgiveness is not just about obedience; it's about reflecting the character of God in our relationships.

Forgiveness is a powerful tool in your spiritual journey. It breaks the cycle of hurt, heals wounds, and restores relationships. It also liberates you from the anxiety that can arise from holding onto past hurts. By choosing to forgive, you align yourself with God's will and open your heart to the peace that surpasses all understanding.

**Reflection and Commitment**

As you reflect on this chapter, consider the following questions:

1. **Who in your life do you need to forgive? What steps can you take to begin this process?**

2. **Are there areas where you need to forgive yourself? How can you embrace God's forgiveness and extend it to yourself?**

3. **How has holding onto unforgiveness contributed to your anxiety? How can releasing it bring you closer to peace?**

Write down your reflections and bring them before God in prayer. Ask for His guidance and strength as you work through the process of forgiveness. Remember, forgiveness is not just a one-time act; it's a journey of continual release and renewal.

In the next chapter, we'll explore how to find peace in the present moment, embracing the now with faith and trust in God's plan. As you continue on your journey, know that forgiveness is a key that unlocks the door to freedom from anxiety and a deeper connection with God.

## Chapter 8: Finding Peace in the Present Moment

### Mindfulness and Faith

In a world filled with distractions, stress, and uncertainty, it's easy to become overwhelmed by anxiety about the future or regrets from the past.

These anxieties can pull you away from the peace that is available to you in the present moment. One powerful way to combat this is through the practice of mindfulness—being fully present and engaged in the current moment, grounded in your faith.

Mindfulness, when rooted in faith, is more than just a relaxation technique. It's an intentional focus on God's presence in the here and now. Psalm 46:10 reminds us, "Be still, and know that I am God." This verse calls us to pause, quiet our minds, and recognize God's sovereignty in every moment.

By practicing mindfulness, you can learn to quiet the anxious thoughts that try to dominate your mind. Instead of worrying about the future or dwelling on the past, you can choose to focus on the present and on God's presence in your life. This

shift in focus can bring immediate relief from

anxiety and help you cultivate a deep sense of

peace.

**Living in the Now**

Living in the present moment means embracing the

here and now, trusting that God is with you and that

His grace is sufficient for today. Jesus teaches this

in Matthew 6:34: "Therefore do not worry about

tomorrow, for tomorrow will worry about itself.

Each day has enough trouble of its own." This verse

encourages you to focus on today, knowing that

God will take care of the future.

When you live in the now, you allow yourself to fully experience the blessings and opportunities that each day offers. You become more aware of God's presence in your life and more attuned to the ways He is working around you. This awareness can reduce anxiety, as it shifts your focus from what might happen to what is happening—right now, in this moment.

To practice living in the now, start by paying attention to your daily routines. Whether you're eating a meal, taking a walk, or spending time with loved ones, try to be fully present. Notice the sights, sounds, and sensations around you. As you do, remind yourself that God is with you, in this moment, providing everything you need.

**Scriptures on Peace**

The Bible is rich with verses that speak to the peace that comes from trusting in God and living in the present moment. Here are a few key scriptures to meditate on:

1. **Isaiah 26:3**: "You will keep in perfect peace those whose minds are steadfast, because they trust in you." This verse emphasizes the connection between trusting God and experiencing peace. When your mind is focused on God, you can rest in His peace.

2. **Philippians 4:6-7**: "Do not be anxious about anything, but in every situation, by prayer and petition, with thanksgiving, present your requests to God. And the peace of God,

which transcends all understanding, will guard your hearts and your minds in Christ Jesus." This passage reminds you to bring your anxieties to God in prayer, trusting that His peace will protect you.

3.  **John 14:27**: "Peace I leave with you; my peace I give you. I do not give to you as the world gives. Do not let your hearts be troubled and do not be afraid." Jesus offers His peace as a gift, a peace that is different from what the world offers—one that is deep, lasting, and not dependent on circumstances.

**Practical Techniques for Mindfulness**

Here are some practical techniques to help you incorporate mindfulness and living in the present moment into your daily life:

1. **Breathing Exercises**: Take a few moments each day to practice deep breathing. Focus on your breath as it enters and leaves your body, using this time to center yourself and bring your thoughts back to the present.

2. **Gratitude Practice**: Each day, take a few minutes to reflect on what you are grateful for in the present moment. This practice can shift your focus from anxiety to appreciation, helping you to see the good that is already in your life.

3. **Mindful Prayer**: Incorporate mindfulness
   into your prayer life by focusing on each
   word of your prayers and being fully present
   with God. This can deepen your connection
   with Him and enhance your sense of peace.

4. **Meditation on Scripture**: Choose a verse or
   passage from the Bible and meditate on it,
   allowing its truth to fill your mind and heart.
   This practice can help you stay rooted in
   God's Word throughout the day.

**Reflection and Commitment**

As you reflect on this chapter, consider how you
can bring more mindfulness and present-moment
awareness into your daily life. Ask yourself:

1.  **How often do I find myself worrying about the future or dwelling on the past?**

2.  **What can I do to become more present in my daily activities?**

3.  **How can I incorporate mindfulness and faith into my spiritual practices?**

Write down your reflections and make a commitment to practice living in the now, trusting that God is with you in every moment. As you do, you'll begin to experience the peace that comes from knowing that God is in control, here and now.

In the next chapter, we'll explore how to live fully in the light of faith, integrating these practices into your daily life so that anxiety no longer has power over you. As you continue on this journey, know that each moment is an opportunity to connect with God and embrace His peace.

## Chapter 9: Living in the Light

### Embracing Faith as a Lifestyle

As you've journeyed through the previous chapters, you've begun to understand the importance of faith in overcoming anxiety. But faith is not just something to be called upon in times of need; it's a way of life. Embracing faith as a lifestyle means allowing it to permeate every aspect of your existence, guiding your thoughts, actions, and decisions.

Living in the light of faith is about consistently choosing to trust in God, even when circumstances are challenging. It's about making faith the foundation upon which you build your life, rather than just a tool to use in emergencies. This shift in perspective can bring about profound changes in how you experience the world, reducing anxiety and filling your life with peace.

Consider how you can incorporate faith into your daily routine. Whether it's through prayer, scripture reading, acts of service, or simply being mindful of God's presence throughout your day, these practices can help you live in the light of faith. The more you integrate faith into your life, the less room there is for anxiety to take hold.

**The Peace that Passes Understanding**

One of the most beautiful promises in the Bible is the peace that God offers—a peace that surpasses all human understanding. This peace is not dependent on external circumstances but is rooted in the assurance that God is in control. Philippians 4:6-7 reminds us, "Do not be anxious about anything, but in every situation, by prayer and petition, with thanksgiving, present your requests to God. And the peace of God, which transcends all understanding, will guard your hearts and your minds in Christ Jesus."

This peace is available to you, no matter what challenges you face. It's a peace that can calm the storm within you, even when the world around you is chaotic. By living in the light of faith, you open yourself up to this peace, allowing it to guard your heart and mind against the anxieties that try to intrude.

To experience this peace, make it a habit to turn to God in every situation. When anxiety starts to rise, pause and bring your concerns to Him in prayer. Thank Him for His presence and for the peace that He offers. As you do this consistently, you'll begin to notice a shift—a deep, abiding peace that stays with you, regardless of what's happening around you.

**Spiritual Growth and Transformation**

Living in the light of faith is not just about maintaining peace; it's also about ongoing spiritual growth and transformation. As you continue to walk in faith, you'll find that God is continually shaping you, helping you to become more like Christ. This process of growth can lead to greater resilience, deeper joy, and a stronger sense of purpose.

Romans 12:2 encourages us, "Do not conform to the pattern of this world, but be transformed by the renewing of your mind. Then you will be able to test and approve what God's will is—his good, pleasing and perfect will." This transformation is a lifelong journey, one that involves continually renewing your mind through scripture, prayer, and the guidance of the Holy Spirit.

As you grow spiritually, you'll find that your perspective on anxiety and fear begins to change. What once seemed overwhelming may start to appear as an opportunity for growth. You'll begin to see challenges as chances to deepen your faith, trusting that God is using every experience to mold you into the person He created you to be.

## Stories of Transformation

Hearing stories of how others have been transformed by living in the light of faith can be incredibly encouraging. These testimonies serve as reminders that God is at work in the lives of His people, bringing them from darkness to light, from fear to faith.

Consider reading or listening to testimonies of individuals who have overcome anxiety and fear through their faith. These stories can offer inspiration and hope, showing you that transformation is possible and that you are not alone on this journey.

You might also take time to reflect on your own journey. How have you changed since you began to live in the light of faith? What transformations have you experienced? Sharing your story with others can be a powerful way to encourage and uplift those who are still struggling with anxiety.

**Reflection and Application**

As you reflect on this chapter, consider the following questions:

1. **How can I make faith more central to my daily life, ensuring that it guides all my actions and decisions?**

2. **In what areas of my life have I already experienced the peace that surpasses understanding? How can I cultivate this peace more consistently?**

3. **What steps can I take to continue growing spiritually and allow God to transform my life?**

Take time to write down your reflections and bring them before God in prayer. Ask for His help in living fully in the light of faith, embracing the peace and transformation that He offers.

In the next chapter, we'll explore how to share the light you've found with others, encouraging those around you to embark on their own journeys from fear to faith. As you continue on this path, remember that living in the light is a lifelong journey, one that brings you closer to the heart of God with each step you take.

## Chapter 10: Sharing the Light with Others

**Becoming a Beacon**

As you've walked the path from fear to faith and experienced the peace that comes from living in the light, you now have an opportunity to become a beacon of hope for others. Sharing the light you've found is not only a way to encourage others but also a powerful way to strengthen your own faith. When you share your journey, you reaffirm the truths you've learned and inspire those who may be struggling in darkness.

Jesus calls us to be lights in the world, reflecting His love and truth to those around us. In Matthew 5:14-16, He says, "You are the light of the world. A town built on a hill cannot be hidden. Neither do people light a lamp and put it under a bowl. Instead, they put it on its stand, and it gives light to everyone in the house. In the same way, let your light shine before others, that they may see your good deeds and glorify your Father in heaven.”

As you let your light shine, you bring glory to God and offer others a glimpse of the peace and hope that faith provides. Whether it's through words, actions, or simply the way you live your life, your light has the power to make a difference in the lives of those around you.

**Encouraging Others Who Struggle with Anxiety**

One of the most powerful ways you can share the light is by encouraging others who struggle with anxiety. Because you've walked this path yourself, you understand the challenges and fears that come with anxiety. Your experience gives you a unique ability to empathize and offer support to others who are in the midst of their own battles.

When you encounter someone who is struggling with anxiety, consider how you can offer encouragement and hope. This might involve sharing your own story, offering a listening ear, or providing practical advice on spiritual practices that have helped you. Sometimes, simply being present and reminding them that they are not alone can be a tremendous comfort.

You can also point them to scripture that has brought you peace, praying with them and for them as they navigate their journey. Your presence and support can be a powerful reminder that God is with them, and that there is light even in the darkest of times.

**The Role of Witnessing**

Witnessing is not just about sharing your faith verbally; it's about living in a way that reflects the light of Christ in all you do. Your actions, attitudes, and the way you handle challenges can speak volumes about the power of faith in overcoming anxiety. When others see the peace and joy in your life, they may be drawn to the source of that light.

In 1 Peter 3:15, we are encouraged to "always be prepared to give an answer to everyone who asks you to give the reason for the hope that you have. But do this with gentleness and respect."

Witnessing involves both sharing your story and living in a way that invites others to ask about the hope you have found in Christ.

Be mindful of the opportunities you have to witness through your everyday interactions. Whether it's at work, in your community, or within your family, your life can be a testimony to the transformative power of faith. When others ask how you've found peace or overcome anxiety, be ready to share the hope that comes from trusting in God.

**Building a Faith-Filled Community**

As you continue to share your light with others, consider the importance of building or contributing to a faith-filled community. Being part of a community that supports and encourages one another in faith can provide ongoing strength and inspiration. This community can become a source of light for many, offering hope, support, and a reminder that no one has to journey through life alone.

If you're not already part of a faith community, consider joining a church, small group, or Bible study. These communities can provide you with opportunities to both give and receive support. If you're already involved in a community, think about how you can contribute to its growth and impact, perhaps by starting a group focused on overcoming anxiety through faith or simply by being a source of encouragement to others.

Remember, the light that you share within a community can have a ripple effect, touching the lives of many beyond what you can see. As you invest in others, you're also investing in your own spiritual growth, deepening your faith and strengthening your connection to God.

**Reflection and Application**

As you reflect on this chapter, consider the following questions:

1. **How can I let my light shine more brightly in my everyday life?**

2. **Who in my life could benefit from hearing my story of overcoming anxiety through faith?**

3. **What steps can I take to build or contribute to a faith-filled community that supports and encourages others on their journey from fear to faith?**

Take time to write down your reflections and bring them before God in prayer. Ask Him to guide you as you share your light with others, and trust that He will use your story and your life to impact those around you.

In the final chapter, we'll reflect on the journey you've taken from fear to faith and offer a final encouragement to continue walking in the light, knowing that God's peace and presence are with you always.

# Chapter 11: The Journey Continues

**Facing New Challenges with Faith**

As you reflect on the journey you've taken from fear to faith, it's important to recognize that this journey doesn't end here. Life will continue to bring challenges, uncertainties, and moments of anxiety. However, you now have the tools and spiritual strength to face these challenges with faith, knowing that God is with you every step of the way.

In Isaiah 43:2, God reassures us: "When you pass through the waters, I will be with you; and when you pass through the rivers, they will not sweep over you. When you walk through the fire, you will not be burned; the flames will not set you ablaze." This verse is a powerful reminder that while challenges will come, you are not alone. God's presence is a constant, providing protection, guidance, and peace.

As you continue on your journey, remember to turn to the spiritual practices that have helped you overcome anxiety. Whether it's prayer, scripture reading, worship, or being part of a faith-filled community, these practices will continue to anchor you in God's peace. When new challenges arise, approach them with the confidence that comes from knowing God's light is within you, guiding your path.

## Adapting to Change

Change is a constant in life, and it can often be a source of anxiety. However, by embracing faith, you can view change not as a threat, but as an opportunity for growth and transformation. Ecclesiastes 3:1 reminds us, "There is a time for everything, and a season for every activity under the heavens." This verse speaks to the natural rhythms of life and the understanding that change is a part of God's plan.

When you encounter change, whether it's a new job, a move, a shift in relationships, or something unexpected, approach it with a spirit of openness and trust in God's timing. Remind yourself that God is in control and that He is working all things together for your good (Romans 8:28). By embracing change with faith, you allow God to use these moments to deepen your character and strengthen your reliance on Him.

**Faith as a Lifelong Journey**

The journey from fear to faith is not a destination; it's a lifelong process. Each day presents new opportunities to grow in faith, to trust God more deeply, and to experience His peace in greater measure. As you continue on this journey, it's important to remain committed to your spiritual growth and to keep seeking God in all aspects of your life.

Philippians 3:13-14 encourages us: "Forgetting what is behind and straining toward what is ahead, I press on toward the goal to win the prize for which God has called me heavenward in Christ Jesus." This passage reminds us that faith involves continually moving forward, pressing on toward the goal of living fully in God's presence and purpose.

As you continue to press on, remember that faith is dynamic. It grows, deepens, and evolves as you walk with God. Be patient with yourself in this process, knowing that God is faithfully working in you, shaping you into the person He created you to be.

**A Final Encouragement**

As you conclude this book, take a moment to reflect on how far you've come. You've faced your fears, explored the roots of your anxiety, and learned how to live in the light of faith. You've discovered the power of forgiveness, the importance of living in the present moment, and the joy of sharing your light with others. Most importantly, you've drawn closer to God, who is the true source of peace and strength.

Remember that this journey is ongoing. There will be times when you may stumble, moments when anxiety tries to creep back in. But with the tools and insights you've gained, and with God's constant presence in your life, you have everything you need to overcome these challenges. Keep walking in faith, keep seeking God's light, and trust that He will guide you through whatever comes your way.

In closing, let these words from Proverbs 3:5-6 guide you: "Trust in the Lord with all your heart and lean not on your own understanding; in all your ways submit to him, and he will make your paths straight." Trust in God's guidance, submit your fears and anxieties to Him, and walk confidently in the path He has set before you.

As you continue your journey, may you experience the fullness of God's peace, the depth of His love, and the joy of living in His light.

**Closing Prayer**

Heavenly Father, I thank You for guiding me on this journey from fear to faith. I thank You for the peace that only You can provide, a peace that surpasses all understanding. As I continue on this path, I ask for Your continued presence, strength, and guidance. Help me to trust in You fully, to live in the light of Your love, and to be a beacon of hope for others. May my life reflect Your grace, and may I always find comfort in knowing that You are with me, now and forever. In Jesus' name, I pray. Amen.

## Appendix

## Scripture List: Key Verses for Quick Reference

Here is a list of key scriptures mentioned throughout the book, offering encouragement, strength, and guidance as you continue your journey from fear to faith:

1. **Isaiah 41:10**: "So do not fear, for I am with you; do not be dismayed, for I am your God. I will strengthen you and help you; I will uphold you with my righteous right hand."

2. **Philippians 4:6-7**: "Do not be anxious about anything, but in every situation, by prayer and petition, with thanksgiving, present your requests to God. And the peace of God, which transcends all understanding, will

guard your hearts and your minds in Christ

Jesus."

3.  **Psalm 46:1**: "God is our refuge and

strength, an ever-present help in trouble."

4.  **Matthew 6:34**: "Therefore do not worry

about tomorrow, for tomorrow will worry

about itself. Each day has enough trouble of

its own."

5.  **Proverbs 3:5-6**: "Trust in the Lord with all

your heart and lean not on your own

understanding; in all your ways submit to

him, and he will make your paths straight."

6.  **Isaiah 26:3**: "You will keep in perfect peace

those whose minds are steadfast, because

they trust in you."

7.  **Lamentations 3:25-26**: "The Lord is good to those whose hope is in him, to the one who seeks him; it is good to wait quietly for the salvation of the Lord."

8.  **Romans 8:25**: "But if we hope for what we do not yet have, we wait for it patiently."

9.  **1 Peter 5:7**: "Cast all your anxiety on him because he cares for you."

10. **John 14:27**: "Peace I leave with you; my peace I give you. I do not give to you as the world gives. Do not let your hearts be troubled and do not be afraid."

**Prayers for Peace and Strength**

These prayers are designed to help you find peace and strength in moments of anxiety. Feel free to personalize them as you pray:

**1. Prayer for Calm in the Storm** Heavenly Father, I come to You in the midst of my anxiety, asking for Your calming presence to surround me. Help me to remember that You are in control, even when everything feels chaotic. Fill my heart with Your peace, and guide me through this storm. I trust in You, Lord, and I thank You for Your constant care. In Jesus' name, Amen.

**2. Prayer for Trust in God's Timing** Lord, I admit that I struggle with patience and want things to happen on my timeline. Help me to surrender my need for control and to trust in Your perfect timing.

Teach me to wait with hope, knowing that You are working all things for my good. Strengthen my faith as I rely on Your wisdom. In Jesus' name, Amen.

**3. Prayer for Strength in Weakness** Father God, I feel weak and overwhelmed by the challenges before me. But I know that in my weakness, Your strength is made perfect. Empower me with Your Spirit, and give me the courage to face whatever lies ahead. Remind me that I am never alone, for You are always with me. In Jesus' name, Amen.

**4. Prayer for Peace in the Present Moment**

Gracious God, help me to focus on the present moment and to find peace in Your presence. Still my anxious thoughts and remind me that You are here with me, providing everything I need. Teach me to live in the now, trusting that You hold my future in Your hands. In Jesus' name, Amen.

**5. Prayer for Overcoming Fear** Lord, fear often grips my heart and mind, but I know that You have not given me a spirit of fear, but of power, love, and a sound mind. Help me to cast out fear by focusing on Your love and truth. Fill me with Your courage, and help me to walk confidently in faith. In Jesus' name, Amen.

**Reflection Questions**

Use these reflection questions for deeper study and personal growth. They correspond to the themes of each chapter:

**Chapter 1: The Darkness of Fear**

- What specific fears or anxieties do you struggle with most? How have these fears impacted your life?

- How do you currently respond to fear, and what changes can you make to respond with faith instead?

## Chapter 2: The Roots of Anxiety

- What triggers your anxiety? How are these triggers connected to past experiences or generational patterns?

- What steps can you take to address the roots of your anxiety with God's help?

## Chapter 3: The Light Begins to Shine

- How have you experienced God's presence in the midst of your anxiety?

- What spiritual practices help you stay connected to God's light?

**Chapter 4: Guided by the Light**

- In what areas of your life do you need to trust God more fully? How can you incorporate spiritual practices into your daily routine?

- Who in your life can support you on your journey from fear to faith?

**Chapter 5: Trusting in God's Timing**

- Are there situations where you struggle to trust God's timing? How can you surrender control to Him?

- How can waiting with hope change your perspective on current challenges?

## Chapter 6: Overcoming Obstacles on the Path

- What doubts or obstacles have you faced on your journey? How can scripture help you overcome them?

- What spiritual armor can you put on to resist the darkness and stay strong in faith?

## Chapter 7: The Power of Forgiveness

- Who in your life do you need to forgive? How can releasing resentment bring you peace?

- How can you practice self-forgiveness and accept God's grace in your life?

**Chapter 8: Finding Peace in the Present Moment**

- How often do you find yourself worrying about the future or dwelling on the past?

- What can you do to become more present in your daily activities and trust God's provision for today?

**Chapter 9: Living in the Light**

- How can you make faith more central to your daily life?

- In what ways have you experienced spiritual growth, and how can you continue to grow?

## Chapter 10: Sharing the Light with Others

- How can you let your light shine more brightly in your everyday life?
- Who in your life could benefit from hearing your story of overcoming anxiety through faith?

## Resources

Here are some additional resources that may be helpful as you continue your journey from fear to faith:

## Support Groups

- **Celebrate Recovery**: A Christ-centered recovery program for anyone struggling with hurts, habits, and hang-ups, including anxiety.

- **NAMI (National Alliance on Mental Illness)**: Offers support groups and resources for those struggling with mental health issues, including anxiety.

- **GriefShare**: A support group for those dealing with loss and grief, which can often exacerbate anxiety.

**Online Resources**

- **Focus on the Family**: www.focusonthefamily.com (Offers articles, podcasts, and resources on dealing with anxiety from a Christian perspective.)

- **Christian Counseling & Educational Foundation (CCEF)**: www.ccef.org (Provides resources for biblical counseling and dealing with anxiety.)

- **YouVersion Bible App**: www.youversion.com (Offers Bible reading plans and devotionals focused on overcoming anxiety.)

**Counseling Services**

- **Faithful Counseling**: www.faithfulcounseling.com (Online Christian counseling services.)

- **Christian Counseling & Educational Foundation (CCEF)**: www.ccef.org (Directory of Christian counselors.)

This appendix is designed to provide you with quick access to scriptures, prayers, reflection questions, and resources that can support you in your journey. Use it as a companion to the chapters, returning to it whenever you need encouragement or guidance.

## A Letter from the Author

Dear Reader,

As I write this letter, I find myself reflecting on the journey you've just undertaken through the pages of this book. It's a journey that many of us know all too well—a journey from fear to faith, from anxiety to peace. It's not an easy path, but it's one that is filled with hope, transformation, and the promise of God's unfailing love.

Writing this book has been a deeply personal experience for me. Like you, I have faced moments of anxiety, times when fear seemed overwhelming and peace felt elusive. But through those moments, I've learned that God's light is always shining, even in the darkest of times. It's a light that guides, heals, and restores. My prayer is that this book has helped you to see that light more clearly in your own life.

I want to thank you for allowing me to walk with you on this journey. I know how difficult it can be to confront your fears and to seek peace in the midst of anxiety. But I also know the incredible strength and peace that come when we place our trust in God. You've taken a courageous step by choosing to face your fears and to seek a deeper connection with God. For that, I commend you.

As you move forward, I encourage you to keep the lessons and practices from this book close to your heart. Continue to seek God in every moment—especially in those moments when anxiety threatens to return. Remember that you are never alone; God is always with you, guiding your steps, calming your heart, and filling you with His peace.

Please know that I am praying for you. I pray that you will continue to grow in faith, that you will experience the fullness of God's love, and that you will live each day in the light of His presence. I pray that you will find joy in the journey, even in the midst of challenges, and that you will become a beacon of hope for others who may be struggling.

If this book has touched your life in some way, I would love to hear from you. Your stories, your feedback, and your experiences are important to me. They remind me of the incredible ways that God is at work in all of our lives, drawing us closer to Him.

Thank you, once again, for allowing me to share this journey with you. May God bless you abundantly as you continue to walk in His light.

With faith and gratitude,

Kristine Hawkins,

Author of *From Fear to Faith: Conquering Anxiety*

*with Spiritual Strength*